Ehlers Danlos Syndrome Book

PRESENTED TO FROM DATE

Volume · edition: __ Year: ___

This Book Belongs To

if found, please return to its owner — thank you

This book belongs to: ______________________________

Phone: __________________ Email: __________________

HOME · RETURN ADDRESS

IF FOUND, PLEASE CONTACT

REWARD IF RETURNED

NOTES · IMPORTANT DETAILS

In use from: __________________ To: ______________

Medical Directory

Directory of specialists and providers

EMERGENCY & URGENT CARE NUMBERS

PRIMARY CARE PROVIDER

RHEUMATOLOGIST

GENETICIST

CARDIOLOGIST

PHYSICAL THERAPISTS

OTHER SPECIALISTS

PHARMACY & SUPPLIES

INSURANCE & PORTALS

Medical Directory

Directory of specialists and providers

EMERGENCY & URGENT CARE NUMBERS

PRIMARY CARE PROVIDER

RHEUMATOLOGIST

GENETICIST

CARDIOLOGIST

PHYSICAL THERAPISTS

OTHER SPECIALISTS

PHARMACY & SUPPLIES

INSURANCE & PORTALS

Baseline Assessment

Hypermobility & Comorbidities Tracker

Date: ______________ **Patient / Name:** ________________

BEIGHTON SCORE (MAX 9)

Maneuver	Left (1 pt)	Right (1 pt)	Total

COMORBIDITIES CHECKLIST

- ☐ POTS / Dysautonomia
- ☐ MCAS / Allergies
- ☐ Gastroparesis / GI Issues
- ☐ Chronic Fatigue (ME/CFS)
- ☐ TMJ / Jaw Issues
- ☐ Migraines / Headaches
- ☐ Neuropathy / Nerve Pain

OVERALL PAIN LEVEL: ○○○○○○○○○○

OVERALL FATIGUE: ○○○○○○○○○

PAIN MAP (SHADE OR DESCRIBE AREAS)

PRIMARY SYMPTOMS & TRIGGERS

MANAGEMENT PLAN & NEXT STEPS (REFERRALS, PT, MEDS)

DESCRIPTION

TARGET DATE

WHY THIS MATTERS

ACTION STEPS

PROGRESS:

Baseline Assessment

Hypermobility & Comorbidities Tracker

Date: ______________ **Patient / Name:** ______________

BEIGHTON SCORE (MAX 9)

Maneuver	Left (1 pt)	Right (1 pt)	Total

COMORBIDITIES CHECKLIST

- ☐ POTS / Dysautonomia
- ☐ MCAS / Allergies
- ☐ Gastroparesis / GI Issues
- ☐ Chronic Fatigue (ME/CFS)
- ☐ TMJ / Jaw Issues
- ☐ Migraines / Headaches
- ☐ Neuropathy / Nerve Pain

OVERALL PAIN LEVEL: ○ ○ ○ ○ ○ ○ ○ ○ ○ ○

OVERALL FATIGUE: ○ ○ ○ ○ ○ ○ ○ ○ ○ ○

PAIN MAP (SHADE OR DESCRIBE AREAS)

PRIMARY SYMPTOMS & TRIGGERS

MANAGEMENT PLAN & NEXT STEPS (REFERRALS, PT, MEDS)

DESCRIPTION

TARGET DATE

WHY THIS MATTERS

ACTION STEPS

PROGRESS:

Baseline Assessment

Hypermobility & Comorbidities Tracker

Date: ______________ **Patient / Name:** ______________

BEIGHTON SCORE (MAX 9)

Maneuver	Left (1 pt)	Right (1 pt)	Total

COMORBIDITIES CHECKLIST

- [ ] POTS / Dysautonomia
- [ ] MCAS / Allergies
- [ ] Gastroparesis / GI Issues
- [ ] Chronic Fatigue (ME/CFS)
- [ ] TMJ / Jaw Issues
- [ ] Migraines / Headaches
- [ ] Neuropathy / Nerve Pain

OVERALL PAIN LEVEL: ○○○○○○○○○○

OVERALL FATIGUE: ○○○○○○○

PAIN MAP (SHADE OR DESCRIBE AREAS)

PRIMARY SYMPTOMS & TRIGGERS

MANAGEMENT PLAN & NEXT STEPS (REFERRALS, PT, MEDS)

DESCRIPTION

TARGET DATE

WHY THIS MATTERS

ACTION STEPS

1

PROGRESS:

Baseline Assessment

Hypermobility & Comorbidities Tracker

Date: ____________ **Patient / Name:** ____________

BEIGHTON SCORE (MAX 9)

Maneuver	Left (1 pt)	Right (1 pt)	Total

COMORBIDITIES CHECKLIST

- ☐ POTS / Dysautonomia
- ☐ MCAS / Allergies
- ☐ Gastroparesis / GI Issues
- ☐ Chronic Fatigue (ME/CFS)
- ☐ TMJ / Jaw Issues
- ☐ Migraines / Headaches
- ☐ Neuropathy / Nerve Pain

OVERALL PAIN LEVEL: ○ ○ ○ ○ ○ ○ ○ ○ ○ ○

OVERALL FATIGUE: ○ ○ ○ ○ ○ ○ ○ ○ ○ ○

PAIN MAP (SHADE OR DESCRIBE AREAS)

PRIMARY SYMPTOMS & TRIGGERS

MANAGEMENT PLAN & NEXT STEPS (REFERRALS, PT, MEDS)

DESCRIPTION

TARGET DATE

WHY THIS MATTERS

ACTION STEPS

PROGRESS:

Medication Tracker

Current Prescriptions & Supplements

Patient Name: _____ **Date Updated:** _____ **Dr. / Clinic:** _____

ROUTINE MEDICATIONS & SUPPLEMENTS

Name	Dosage	Frequency / Time	Start Date	Reason / Notes

EMERGENCY & RESCUE MEDICATIONS (AS NEEDED)

Medication	Dosage	When to use / Symptoms	Exp. Date

PHARMACY INFO, REFILL DATES & ADDITIONAL NOTES

Medication Tracker

Current Prescriptions & Supplements

Patient Name: ______ **Date Updated:** ______ **Dr. / Clinic:** ______

ROUTINE MEDICATIONS & SUPPLEMENTS

Name	Dosage	Frequency / Time	Start Date	Reason / Notes

EMERGENCY & RESCUE MEDICATIONS (AS NEEDED)

Medication	Dosage	When to use / Symptoms	Exp. Date

PHARMACY INFO, REFILL DATES & ADDITIONAL NOTES

Medication Tracker

Current Prescriptions & Supplements

Patient Name: ______ **Date Updated:** ______ **Dr. / Clinic:** ______

ROUTINE MEDICATIONS & SUPPLEMENTS

Name	Dosage	Frequency / Time	Start Date	Reason / Notes

EMERGENCY & RESCUE MEDICATIONS (AS NEEDED)

Medication	Dosage	When to use / Symptoms	Exp. Date

PHARMACY INFO, REFILL DATES & ADDITIONAL NOTES

Medication Tracker

Current Prescriptions & Supplements

Patient Name: _____ **Date Updated:** _____ **Dr. / Clinic:** _____

ROUTINE MEDICATIONS & SUPPLEMENTS

Name	Dosage	Frequency / Time	Start Date	Reason / Notes

EMERGENCY & RESCUE MEDICATIONS (AS NEEDED)

Medication	Dosage	When to use / Symptoms	Exp. Date

PHARMACY INFO, REFILL DATES & ADDITIONAL NOTES

Monthly Health Overview

Pain, fatigue, cycle, and environmental tracking

Month / Year: _________ Monthly Focus / Goal: ______

SYMPTOM & CYCLE CALENDAR (COLOR-CODE PAIN, FATIGUE, AND CYCLE DAYS)

S	M	T	W	T	F	S

BAROMETRIC & WEATHER SHIFTS

Date	Weather / Pressure Shift	Symptom Impact

COLOR LEGEND & SCALES

FLARE & PAIN NOTES

CYCLE & FATIGUE NOTES

Monthly Health Overview

Pain, fatigue, cycle, and environmental tracking

Month / Year: _________ Monthly Focus / Goal: ______

SYMPTOM & CYCLE CALENDAR (COLOR-CODE PAIN, FATIGUE, AND CYCLE DAYS)

S	M	T	W	T	F	S

BAROMETRIC & WEATHER SHIFTS

Date	Weather / Pressure Shift	Symptom Impact

COLOR LEGEND & SCALES

FLARE & PAIN NOTES

CYCLE & FATIGUE NOTES

Monthly Health Overview

Pain, fatigue, cycle, and environmental tracking

Month / Year: _________ Monthly Focus / Goal: ______

SYMPTOM & CYCLE CALENDAR (COLOR-CODE PAIN, FATIGUE, AND CYCLE DAYS)

S	M	T	W	T	F	S

BAROMETRIC & WEATHER SHIFTS

Date	Weather / Pressure Shift	Symptom Impact

COLOR LEGEND & SCALES

FLARE & PAIN NOTES

CYCLE & FATIGUE NOTES

Monthly Health Overview

Pain, fatigue, cycle, and environmental tracking

Month / Year: _________ Monthly Focus / Goal: _______

SYMPTOM & CYCLE CALENDAR (COLOR-CODE PAIN, FATIGUE, AND CYCLE DAYS)

S	M	T	W	T	F	S

BAROMETRIC & WEATHER SHIFTS

Date	Weather / Pressure Shift	Symptom Impact

COLOR LEGEND & SCALES

FLARE & PAIN NOTES

CYCLE & FATIGUE NOTES

Monthly Health Overview

Pain, fatigue, cycle, and environmental tracking

Month / Year: __________   Monthly Focus / Goal: ________

SYMPTOM & CYCLE CALENDAR (COLOR-CODE PAIN, FATIGUE, AND CYCLE DAYS)

S	M	T	W	T	F	S

BAROMETRIC & WEATHER SHIFTS

Date	Weather / Pressure Shift	Symptom Impact

COLOR LEGEND & SCALES

FLARE & PAIN NOTES

CYCLE & FATIGUE NOTES

Monthly Health Overview

Pain, fatigue, cycle, and environmental tracking

Month / Year: _________ **Monthly Focus / Goal:** _______

SYMPTOM & CYCLE CALENDAR (COLOR-CODE PAIN, FATIGUE, AND CYCLE DAYS)

S	M	T	W	T	F	S

BAROMETRIC & WEATHER SHIFTS

Date	Weather / Pressure Shift	Symptom Impact

COLOR LEGEND & SCALES

FLARE & PAIN NOTES

CYCLE & FATIGUE NOTES

Weekly Symptom Log

Part 1: Monday - Thursday

Week of: ________

Mon: _____ PAIN: ☐☐☐☐☐☐☐☐☐☐ FATIGUE: ☐☐☐☐☐☐☐☐☐☐ BRAIN FOG: ☐☐☐☐☐☐☐☐☐☐

JOINTS SUBLUXATED / DISLOCATED

Tue: _____ PAIN: ☐☐☐☐☐☐☐☐☐☐ FATIGUE: ☐☐☐☐☐☐☐☐☐☐ BRAIN FOG: ☐☐☐☐☐☐☐☐☐☐

JOINTS SUBLUXATED / DISLOCATED

Wed: _____ PAIN: ☐☐☐☐☐☐☐☐☐☐ FATIGUE: ☐☐☐☐☐☐☐☐☐☐ BRAIN FOG: ☐☐☐☐☐☐☐☐☐☐

JOINTS SUBLUXATED / DISLOCATED

Thu: _____ PAIN: ☐☐☐☐☐☐☐☐☐☐ FATIGUE: ☐☐☐☐☐☐☐☐☐☐ BRAIN FOG: ☐☐☐☐☐☐☐☐☐☐

JOINTS SUBLUXATED / DISLOCATED

MEDICATION ADJUSTMENTS & GENERAL NOTES

Weekly Symptom Log

Part 1: Monday - Thursday

Week of: __________

Mon: ______ PAIN: ☐☐☐☐☐☐☐☐☐☐ FATIGUE: ☐☐☐☐☐☐☐☐☐☐ BRAIN FOG: ☐☐☐☐☐☐☐☐☐☐

JOINTS SUBLUXATED / DISLOCATED

Tue: ______ PAIN: ☐☐☐☐☐☐☐☐☐☐ FATIGUE: ☐☐☐☐☐☐☐☐☐☐ BRAIN FOG: ☐☐☐☐☐☐☐☐☐☐

JOINTS SUBLUXATED / DISLOCATED

Wed: ______ PAIN: ☐☐☐☐☐☐☐☐☐☐ FATIGUE: ☐☐☐☐☐☐☐☐☐☐ BRAIN FOG: ☐☐☐☐☐☐☐☐☐☐

JOINTS SUBLUXATED / DISLOCATED

Thu: ______ PAIN: ☐☐☐☐☐☐☐☐☐☐ FATIGUE: ☐☐☐☐☐☐☐☐☐☐ BRAIN FOG: ☐☐☐☐☐☐☐☐☐☐

JOINTS SUBLUXATED / DISLOCATED

MEDICATION ADJUSTMENTS & GENERAL NOTES

Weekly Symptom Log

Part 1: Monday - Thursday

Week of: ________

Mon: _____ PAIN: FATIGUE: BRAIN FOG:

JOINTS SUBLUXATED / DISLOCATED

Tue: _____ PAIN: FATIGUE: BRAIN FOG:

JOINTS SUBLUXATED / DISLOCATED

Wed: _____ PAIN: FATIGUE: BRAIN FOG:

JOINTS SUBLUXATED / DISLOCATED

Thu: _____ PAIN: FATIGUE: BRAIN FOG:

JOINTS SUBLUXATED / DISLOCATED

MEDICATION ADJUSTMENTS & GENERAL NOTES

Weekly Symptom Log
Part 1: Monday - Thursday

Week of: ________

Mon: _____ PAIN: ☐☐☐☐☐☐☐☐☐☐ FATIGUE: ☐☐☐☐☐☐☐☐☐☐ BRAIN FOG: ☐☐☐☐☐☐☐☐☐☐

JOINTS SUBLUXATED / DISLOCATED

Tue: _____ PAIN: ☐☐☐☐☐☐☐☐☐☐ FATIGUE: ☐☐☐☐☐☐☐☐☐☐ BRAIN FOG: ☐☐☐☐☐☐☐☐☐☐

JOINTS SUBLUXATED / DISLOCATED

Wed: _____ PAIN: ☐☐☐☐☐☐☐☐☐☐ FATIGUE: ☐☐☐☐☐☐☐☐☐☐ BRAIN FOG: ☐☐☐☐☐☐☐☐☐☐

JOINTS SUBLUXATED / DISLOCATED

Thu: _____ PAIN: ☐☐☐☐☐☐☐☐☐☐ FATIGUE: ☐☐☐☐☐☐☐☐☐☐ BRAIN FOG: ☐☐☐☐☐☐☐☐☐☐

JOINTS SUBLUXATED / DISLOCATED

MEDICATION ADJUSTMENTS & GENERAL NOTES

Weekly Symptom Log
Part 1: Monday - Thursday

Week of: ________

Mon: _____ PAIN: FATIGUE: BRAIN FOG:

JOINTS SUBLUXATED / DISLOCATED

Tue: _____ PAIN: FATIGUE: BRAIN FOG:

JOINTS SUBLUXATED / DISLOCATED

Wed: _____ PAIN: FATIGUE: BRAIN FOG:

JOINTS SUBLUXATED / DISLOCATED

Thu: _____ PAIN: FATIGUE: BRAIN FOG:

JOINTS SUBLUXATED / DISLOCATED

MEDICATION ADJUSTMENTS & GENERAL NOTES

Weekly Symptom Log
Part 1: Monday - Thursday

Week of: ________

Mon: _____ PAIN: FATIGUE: BRAIN FOG:

JOINTS SUBLUXATED / DISLOCATED

Tue: _____ PAIN: FATIGUE: BRAIN FOG:

JOINTS SUBLUXATED / DISLOCATED

Wed: _____ PAIN: FATIGUE: BRAIN FOG:

JOINTS SUBLUXATED / DISLOCATED

Thu: _____ PAIN: FATIGUE: BRAIN FOG:

JOINTS SUBLUXATED / DISLOCATED

MEDICATION ADJUSTMENTS & GENERAL NOTES

Weekly Symptom Log

Part 1: Monday - Thursday

Week of: ________

Mon: _____ PAIN: ☐☐☐☐☐☐☐☐☐☐ FATIGUE: ☐☐☐☐☐☐☐☐☐☐ BRAIN FOG: ☐☐☐☐☐☐☐☐☐☐

JOINTS SUBLUXATED / DISLOCATED

Tue: _____ PAIN: ☐☐☐☐☐☐☐☐☐☐ FATIGUE: ☐☐☐☐☐☐☐☐☐☐ BRAIN FOG: ☐☐☐☐☐☐☐☐☐☐

JOINTS SUBLUXATED / DISLOCATED

Wed: _____ PAIN: ☐☐☐☐☐☐☐☐☐☐ FATIGUE: ☐☐☐☐☐☐☐☐☐☐ BRAIN FOG: ☐☐☐☐☐☐☐☐☐☐

JOINTS SUBLUXATED / DISLOCATED

Thu: _____ PAIN: ☐☐☐☐☐☐☐☐☐☐ FATIGUE: ☐☐☐☐☐☐☐☐☐☐ BRAIN FOG: ☐☐☐☐☐☐☐☐☐☐

JOINTS SUBLUXATED / DISLOCATED

MEDICATION ADJUSTMENTS & GENERAL NOTES

Weekly Symptom Log

Part 1: Monday - Thursday

Week of: ________

Mon: _____ PAIN: FATIGUE: BRAIN FOG:

JOINTS SUBLUXATED / DISLOCATED

Tue: _____ PAIN: FATIGUE: BRAIN FOG:

JOINTS SUBLUXATED / DISLOCATED

Wed: _____ PAIN: FATIGUE: BRAIN FOG:

JOINTS SUBLUXATED / DISLOCATED

Thu: _____ PAIN: FATIGUE: BRAIN FOG:

JOINTS SUBLUXATED / DISLOCATED

MEDICATION ADJUSTMENTS & GENERAL NOTES

Weekly Symptom Log

Part 1: Monday - Thursday

Week of: ________

Mon: _____ PAIN: FATIGUE: BRAIN FOG:

JOINTS SUBLUXATED / DISLOCATED

Tue: _____ PAIN: FATIGUE: BRAIN FOG:

JOINTS SUBLUXATED / DISLOCATED

Wed: _____ PAIN: FATIGUE: BRAIN FOG:

JOINTS SUBLUXATED / DISLOCATED

Thu: _____ PAIN: FATIGUE: BRAIN FOG:

JOINTS SUBLUXATED / DISLOCATED

MEDICATION ADJUSTMENTS & GENERAL NOTES

Weekly Symptom Log

Part 1: Monday - Thursday

Week of: ________

Mon: _____ PAIN: FATIGUE: BRAIN FOG:

JOINTS SUBLUXATED / DISLOCATED

Tue: _____ PAIN: FATIGUE: BRAIN FOG:

JOINTS SUBLUXATED / DISLOCATED

Wed: _____ PAIN: FATIGUE: BRAIN FOG:

JOINTS SUBLUXATED / DISLOCATED

Thu: _____ PAIN: FATIGUE: BRAIN FOG:

JOINTS SUBLUXATED / DISLOCATED

MEDICATION ADJUSTMENTS & GENERAL NOTES

Weekly Symptom Log

Part 1: Monday - Thursday

Week of: ________

Mon: _____ PAIN: ☐☐☐☐☐☐☐☐☐☐ FATIGUE: ☐☐☐☐☐☐☐☐☐☐ BRAIN FOG: ☐☐☐☐☐☐☐☐☐☐

JOINTS SUBLUXATED / DISLOCATED

Tue: _____ PAIN: ☐☐☐☐☐☐☐☐☐☐ FATIGUE: ☐☐☐☐☐☐☐☐☐☐ BRAIN FOG: ☐☐☐☐☐☐☐☐☐☐

JOINTS SUBLUXATED / DISLOCATED

Wed: _____ PAIN: ☐☐☐☐☐☐☐☐☐☐ FATIGUE: ☐☐☐☐☐☐☐☐☐☐ BRAIN FOG: ☐☐☐☐☐☐☐☐☐☐

JOINTS SUBLUXATED / DISLOCATED

Thu: _____ PAIN: ☐☐☐☐☐☐☐☐☐☐ FATIGUE: ☐☐☐☐☐☐☐☐☐☐ BRAIN FOG: ☐☐☐☐☐☐☐☐☐☐

JOINTS SUBLUXATED / DISLOCATED

MEDICATION ADJUSTMENTS & GENERAL NOTES

Weekly Symptom Log

Part 1: Monday - Thursday

Week of: ________

Mon: _____ PAIN: FATIGUE: BRAIN FOG:

JOINTS SUBLUXATED / DISLOCATED

Tue: _____ PAIN: FATIGUE: BRAIN FOG:

JOINTS SUBLUXATED / DISLOCATED

Wed: _____ PAIN: FATIGUE: BRAIN FOG:

JOINTS SUBLUXATED / DISLOCATED

Thu: _____ PAIN: FATIGUE: BRAIN FOG:

JOINTS SUBLUXATED / DISLOCATED

MEDICATION ADJUSTMENTS & GENERAL NOTES

Weekly Symptom Log
Part 1: Monday - Thursday

Week of: ________

Mon: _____ PAIN: FATIGUE: BRAIN FOG:

JOINTS SUBLUXATED / DISLOCATED

Tue: _____ PAIN: FATIGUE: BRAIN FOG:

JOINTS SUBLUXATED / DISLOCATED

Wed: _____ PAIN: FATIGUE: BRAIN FOG:

JOINTS SUBLUXATED / DISLOCATED

Thu: _____ PAIN: FATIGUE: BRAIN FOG:

JOINTS SUBLUXATED / DISLOCATED

MEDICATION ADJUSTMENTS & GENERAL NOTES

Weekly Symptom Log

Part 1: Monday - Thursday

Week of: ________

Mon: _____ PAIN: FATIGUE: BRAIN FOG:

JOINTS SUBLUXATED / DISLOCATED

Tue: _____ PAIN: FATIGUE: BRAIN FOG:

JOINTS SUBLUXATED / DISLOCATED

Wed: _____ PAIN: FATIGUE: BRAIN FOG:

JOINTS SUBLUXATED / DISLOCATED

Thu: _____ PAIN: FATIGUE: BRAIN FOG:

JOINTS SUBLUXATED / DISLOCATED

MEDICATION ADJUSTMENTS & GENERAL NOTES

Weekly Symptom Log

Part 1: Monday - Thursday

Week of: ________

Mon: _____ PAIN: FATIGUE: BRAIN FOG:

JOINTS SUBLUXATED / DISLOCATED

Tue: _____ PAIN: FATIGUE: BRAIN FOG:

JOINTS SUBLUXATED / DISLOCATED

Wed: _____ PAIN: FATIGUE: BRAIN FOG:

JOINTS SUBLUXATED / DISLOCATED

Thu: _____ PAIN: FATIGUE: BRAIN FOG:

JOINTS SUBLUXATED / DISLOCATED

MEDICATION ADJUSTMENTS & GENERAL NOTES

Weekly Symptom Log

Part 1: Monday - Thursday

Week of: ________

Mon: _____ PAIN: FATIGUE: BRAIN FOG:

JOINTS SUBLUXATED / DISLOCATED

Tue: _____ PAIN: FATIGUE: BRAIN FOG:

JOINTS SUBLUXATED / DISLOCATED

Wed: _____ PAIN: FATIGUE: BRAIN FOG:

JOINTS SUBLUXATED / DISLOCATED

Thu: _____ PAIN: FATIGUE: BRAIN FOG:

JOINTS SUBLUXATED / DISLOCATED

MEDICATION ADJUSTMENTS & GENERAL NOTES

Weekly Symptom Log

Part 1: Monday - Thursday

Week of: ________

Mon: _____ PAIN: ☐☐☐☐☐☐☐☐☐☐ FATIGUE: ☐☐☐☐☐☐☐☐☐☐ BRAIN FOG: ☐☐☐☐☐☐☐☐☐☐

JOINTS SUBLUXATED / DISLOCATED

Tue: _____ PAIN: ☐☐☐☐☐☐☐☐☐☐ FATIGUE: ☐☐☐☐☐☐☐☐☐☐ BRAIN FOG: ☐☐☐☐☐☐☐☐☐☐

JOINTS SUBLUXATED / DISLOCATED

Wed: _____ PAIN: ☐☐☐☐☐☐☐☐☐☐ FATIGUE: ☐☐☐☐☐☐☐☐☐☐ BRAIN FOG: ☐☐☐☐☐☐☐☐☐☐

JOINTS SUBLUXATED / DISLOCATED

Thu: _____ PAIN: ☐☐☐☐☐☐☐☐☐☐ FATIGUE: ☐☐☐☐☐☐☐☐☐☐ BRAIN FOG: ☐☐☐☐☐☐☐☐☐☐

JOINTS SUBLUXATED / DISLOCATED

MEDICATION ADJUSTMENTS & GENERAL NOTES

Weekly Symptom Log

Part 1: Monday - Thursday

Week of: ________

Mon: _____ PAIN: ☐☐☐☐☐☐☐☐☐☐ FATIGUE: ☐☐☐☐☐☐☐☐☐☐ BRAIN FOG: ☐☐☐☐☐☐☐☐☐☐

JOINTS SUBLUXATED / DISLOCATED

Tue: _____ PAIN: ☐☐☐☐☐☐☐☐☐☐ FATIGUE: ☐☐☐☐☐☐☐☐☐☐ BRAIN FOG: ☐☐☐☐☐☐☐☐☐☐

JOINTS SUBLUXATED / DISLOCATED

Wed: _____ PAIN: ☐☐☐☐☐☐☐☐☐☐ FATIGUE: ☐☐☐☐☐☐☐☐☐☐ BRAIN FOG: ☐☐☐☐☐☐☐☐☐☐

JOINTS SUBLUXATED / DISLOCATED

Thu: _____ PAIN: ☐☐☐☐☐☐☐☐☐☐ FATIGUE: ☐☐☐☐☐☐☐☐☐☐ BRAIN FOG: ☐☐☐☐☐☐☐☐☐☐

JOINTS SUBLUXATED / DISLOCATED

MEDICATION ADJUSTMENTS & GENERAL NOTES

Weekly Symptom Log

Part 1: Monday - Thursday

Week of: ________

Mon: _____ PAIN: ☐☐☐☐☐☐☐☐☐☐ FATIGUE: ☐☐☐☐☐☐☐☐☐☐ BRAIN FOG: ☐☐☐☐☐☐☐☐☐☐

JOINTS SUBLUXATED / DISLOCATED

Tue: _____ PAIN: ☐☐☐☐☐☐☐☐☐☐ FATIGUE: ☐☐☐☐☐☐☐☐☐☐ BRAIN FOG: ☐☐☐☐☐☐☐☐☐☐

JOINTS SUBLUXATED / DISLOCATED

Wed: _____ PAIN: ☐☐☐☐☐☐☐☐☐☐ FATIGUE: ☐☐☐☐☐☐☐☐☐☐ BRAIN FOG: ☐☐☐☐☐☐☐☐☐☐

JOINTS SUBLUXATED / DISLOCATED

Thu: _____ PAIN: ☐☐☐☐☐☐☐☐☐☐ FATIGUE: ☐☐☐☐☐☐☐☐☐☐ BRAIN FOG: ☐☐☐☐☐☐☐☐☐☐

JOINTS SUBLUXATED / DISLOCATED

MEDICATION ADJUSTMENTS & GENERAL NOTES

Weekly Symptom Log

Part 1: Monday - Thursday

Week of: ________

Mon: _____ PAIN: ☐☐☐☐☐☐☐☐☐☐ FATIGUE: ☐☐☐☐☐☐☐☐☐☐ BRAIN FOG: ☐☐☐☐☐☐☐☐☐☐

JOINTS SUBLUXATED / DISLOCATED

Tue: _____ PAIN: ☐☐☐☐☐☐☐☐☐☐ FATIGUE: ☐☐☐☐☐☐☐☐☐☐ BRAIN FOG: ☐☐☐☐☐☐☐☐☐☐

JOINTS SUBLUXATED / DISLOCATED

Wed: _____ PAIN: ☐☐☐☐☐☐☐☐☐☐ FATIGUE: ☐☐☐☐☐☐☐☐☐☐ BRAIN FOG: ☐☐☐☐☐☐☐☐☐☐

JOINTS SUBLUXATED / DISLOCATED

Thu: _____ PAIN: ☐☐☐☐☐☐☐☐☐☐ FATIGUE: ☐☐☐☐☐☐☐☐☐☐ BRAIN FOG: ☐☐☐☐☐☐☐☐☐☐

JOINTS SUBLUXATED / DISLOCATED

MEDICATION ADJUSTMENTS & GENERAL NOTES

Weekly Symptom Log

Part 1: Monday - Thursday

Week of: ________

Mon: _____ PAIN: ☐ FATIGUE: ☐ BRAIN FOG: ☐

JOINTS SUBLUXATED / DISLOCATED

Tue: _____ PAIN: ☐ FATIGUE: ☐ BRAIN FOG: ☐

JOINTS SUBLUXATED / DISLOCATED

Wed: _____ PAIN: ☐ FATIGUE: ☐ BRAIN FOG: ☐

JOINTS SUBLUXATED / DISLOCATED

Thu: _____ PAIN: ☐ FATIGUE: ☐ BRAIN FOG: ☐

JOINTS SUBLUXATED / DISLOCATED

MEDICATION ADJUSTMENTS & GENERAL NOTES

Weekly Symptom Log

Part 1: Monday - Thursday

Week of: ________

Mon: _____ PAIN: FATIGUE: BRAIN FOG:

JOINTS SUBLUXATED / DISLOCATED

Tue: _____ PAIN: FATIGUE: BRAIN FOG:

JOINTS SUBLUXATED / DISLOCATED

Wed: _____ PAIN: FATIGUE: BRAIN FOG:

JOINTS SUBLUXATED / DISLOCATED

Thu: _____ PAIN: FATIGUE: BRAIN FOG:

JOINTS SUBLUXATED / DISLOCATED

MEDICATION ADJUSTMENTS & GENERAL NOTES

Weekly Symptom Log

Part 1: Monday - Thursday

Week of: ________

Mon: ______ PAIN: FATIGUE: BRAIN FOG:

JOINTS SUBLUXATED / DISLOCATED

Tue: ______ PAIN: FATIGUE: BRAIN FOG:

JOINTS SUBLUXATED / DISLOCATED

Wed: ______ PAIN: FATIGUE: BRAIN FOG:

JOINTS SUBLUXATED / DISLOCATED

Thu: ______ PAIN: FATIGUE: BRAIN FOG:

JOINTS SUBLUXATED / DISLOCATED

MEDICATION ADJUSTMENTS & GENERAL NOTES

Weekly Symptom Log

Part 1: Monday - Thursday

Week of: ________

Mon: _____ PAIN: [ ] FATIGUE: [ ] BRAIN FOG: [ ]

JOINTS SUBLUXATED / DISLOCATED

Tue: _____ PAIN: [ ] FATIGUE: [ ] BRAIN FOG: [ ]

JOINTS SUBLUXATED / DISLOCATED

Wed: _____ PAIN: [ ] FATIGUE: [ ] BRAIN FOG: [ ]

JOINTS SUBLUXATED / DISLOCATED

Thu: _____ PAIN: [ ] FATIGUE: [ ] BRAIN FOG: [ ]

JOINTS SUBLUXATED / DISLOCATED

MEDICATION ADJUSTMENTS & GENERAL NOTES

Weekly Symptom Log
Part 1: Monday - Thursday

Week of: ________

Mon: _____ PAIN: ☐☐☐☐☐☐☐☐☐☐ FATIGUE: ☐☐☐☐☐☐☐☐☐☐ BRAIN FOG: ☐☐☐☐☐☐☐☐☐☐

JOINTS SUBLUXATED / DISLOCATED

Tue: _____ PAIN: ☐☐☐☐☐☐☐☐☐☐ FATIGUE: ☐☐☐☐☐☐☐☐☐☐ BRAIN FOG: ☐☐☐☐☐☐☐☐☐☐

JOINTS SUBLUXATED / DISLOCATED

Wed: _____ PAIN: ☐☐☐☐☐☐☐☐☐☐ FATIGUE: ☐☐☐☐☐☐☐☐☐☐ BRAIN FOG: ☐☐☐☐☐☐☐☐☐☐

JOINTS SUBLUXATED / DISLOCATED

Thu: _____ PAIN: ☐☐☐☐☐☐☐☐☐☐ FATIGUE: ☐☐☐☐☐☐☐☐☐☐ BRAIN FOG: ☐☐☐☐☐☐☐☐☐☐

JOINTS SUBLUXATED / DISLOCATED

MEDICATION ADJUSTMENTS & GENERAL NOTES

Weekly Symptom Log

Part 1: Monday - Thursday

Week of: ________

Mon: _____ PAIN: FATIGUE: BRAIN FOG:

JOINTS SUBLUXATED / DISLOCATED

Tue: _____ PAIN: FATIGUE: BRAIN FOG:

JOINTS SUBLUXATED / DISLOCATED

Wed: _____ PAIN: FATIGUE: BRAIN FOG:

JOINTS SUBLUXATED / DISLOCATED

Thu: _____ PAIN: FATIGUE: BRAIN FOG:

JOINTS SUBLUXATED / DISLOCATED

MEDICATION ADJUSTMENTS & GENERAL NOTES

Weekly Trackers & Notes

Trackers, triggers, and small victories

DAILY PROTOCOLS & METRICS

Hydration Target Met	
Sodium Intake Managed	
Bracing & Taping Applied	
Sleep Quality (Restful)	

TRIGGERS & OBSERVATIONS

SMALL VICTORIES

- [ ]
- [ ]
- [ ]
- [ ]
- [ ]
- [ ]
- [ ]
- [ ]
- [ ]
- [ ]
- [ ]
- [ ]

Weekly Trackers & Notes

Trackers, triggers, and small victories

DAILY PROTOCOLS & METRICS

Hydration Target Met	
Sodium Intake Managed	
Bracing & Taping Applied	
Sleep Quality (Restful)	

TRIGGERS & OBSERVATIONS

SMALL VICTORIES

- [ ]
- [ ]
- [ ]
- [ ]
- [ ]
- [ ]
- [ ]
- [ ]
- [ ]
- [ ]
- [ ]
- [ ]

Weekly Trackers & Notes

Trackers, triggers, and small victories

DAILY PROTOCOLS & METRICS

Hydration Target Met	
Sodium Intake Managed	
Bracing & Taping Applied	
Sleep Quality (Restful)	

TRIGGERS & OBSERVATIONS

SMALL VICTORIES

- [ ]
- [ ]
- [ ]
- [ ]
- [ ]
- [ ]
- [ ]
- [ ]
- [ ]
- [ ]
- [ ]
- [ ]

Weekly Trackers & Notes

Trackers, triggers, and small victories

DAILY PROTOCOLS & METRICS

Hydration Target Met	
Sodium Intake Managed	
Bracing & Taping Applied	
Sleep Quality (Restful)	

TRIGGERS & OBSERVATIONS

SMALL VICTORIES

- [ ]
- [ ]
- [ ]
- [ ]
- [ ]
- [ ]
- [ ]
- [ ]
- [ ]
- [ ]
- [ ]
- [ ]

Weekly Trackers & Notes

Trackers, triggers, and small victories

DAILY PROTOCOLS & METRICS

Hydration Target Met	
Sodium Intake Managed	
Bracing & Taping Applied	
Sleep Quality (Restful)	

TRIGGERS & OBSERVATIONS

SMALL VICTORIES

- [ ]
- [ ]
- [ ]
- [ ]
- [ ]
- [ ]
- [ ]
- [ ]
- [ ]
- [ ]
- [ ]
- [ ]

Weekly Trackers & Notes

Trackers, triggers, and small victories

DAILY PROTOCOLS & METRICS

Hydration Target Met	
Sodium Intake Managed	
Bracing & Taping Applied	
Sleep Quality (Restful)	

TRIGGERS & OBSERVATIONS

SMALL VICTORIES

- [ ]
- [ ]
- [ ]
- [ ]
- [ ]
- [ ]
- [ ]
- [ ]
- [ ]
- [ ]
- [ ]
- [ ]

Weekly Trackers & Notes

Trackers, triggers, and small victories

DAILY PROTOCOLS & METRICS

Hydration Target Met	
Sodium Intake Managed	
Bracing & Taping Applied	
Sleep Quality (Restful)	

TRIGGERS & OBSERVATIONS

SMALL VICTORIES

- [ ]
- [ ]
- [ ]
- [ ]
- [ ]
- [ ]
- [ ]
- [ ]
- [ ]
- [ ]
- [ ]
- [ ]

Weekly Trackers & Notes

Trackers, triggers, and small victories

DAILY PROTOCOLS & METRICS

Hydration Target Met	
Sodium Intake Managed	
Bracing & Taping Applied	
Sleep Quality (Restful)	

TRIGGERS & OBSERVATIONS

SMALL VICTORIES

- [ ]
- [ ]
- [ ]
- [ ]
- [ ]
- [ ]
- [ ]
- [ ]
- [ ]
- [ ]
- [ ]
- [ ]

Weekly Trackers & Notes

Trackers, triggers, and small victories

DAILY PROTOCOLS & METRICS

Hydration Target Met	
Sodium Intake Managed	
Bracing & Taping Applied	
Sleep Quality (Restful)	

TRIGGERS & OBSERVATIONS

SMALL VICTORIES

- [ ]
- [ ]
- [ ]
- [ ]
- [ ]
- [ ]
- [ ]
- [ ]
- [ ]
- [ ]
- [ ]
- [ ]

Weekly Trackers & Notes

Trackers, triggers, and small victories

DAILY PROTOCOLS & METRICS

Hydration Target Met	
Sodium Intake Managed	
Bracing & Taping Applied	
Sleep Quality (Restful)	

TRIGGERS & OBSERVATIONS

SMALL VICTORIES

- [ ]
- [ ]
- [ ]
- [ ]
- [ ]
- [ ]
- [ ]
- [ ]
- [ ]
- [ ]
- [ ]
- [ ]

Weekly Trackers & Notes

Trackers, triggers, and small victories

DAILY PROTOCOLS & METRICS

Hydration Target Met	
Sodium Intake Managed	
Bracing & Taping Applied	
Sleep Quality (Restful)	

TRIGGERS & OBSERVATIONS

SMALL VICTORIES

- [ ]
- [ ]
- [ ]
- [ ]
- [ ]
- [ ]
- [ ]
- [ ]
- [ ]
- [ ]
- [ ]
- [ ]

Weekly Trackers & Notes

Trackers, triggers, and small victories

DAILY PROTOCOLS & METRICS

Hydration Target Met	
Sodium Intake Managed	
Bracing & Taping Applied	
Sleep Quality (Restful)	

TRIGGERS & OBSERVATIONS

SMALL VICTORIES

- [ ]
- [ ]
- [ ]
- [ ]
- [ ]
- [ ]
- [ ]
- [ ]
- [ ]
- [ ]
- [ ]
- [ ]

Weekly Trackers & Notes

Trackers, triggers, and small victories

DAILY PROTOCOLS & METRICS

Hydration Target Met	
Sodium Intake Managed	
Bracing & Taping Applied	
Sleep Quality (Restful)	

TRIGGERS & OBSERVATIONS

SMALL VICTORIES

- [ ]
- [ ]
- [ ]
- [ ]
- [ ]
- [ ]
- [ ]
- [ ]
- [ ]
- [ ]
- [ ]
- [ ]

Weekly Trackers & Notes

Trackers, triggers, and small victories

DAILY PROTOCOLS & METRICS

Hydration Target Met	
Sodium Intake Managed	
Bracing & Taping Applied	
Sleep Quality (Restful)	

TRIGGERS & OBSERVATIONS

SMALL VICTORIES

- [ ]
- [ ]
- [ ]
- [ ]
- [ ]
- [ ]
- [ ]
- [ ]
- [ ]
- [ ]
- [ ]
- [ ]

Weekly Trackers & Notes

Trackers, triggers, and small victories

DAILY PROTOCOLS & METRICS

Hydration Target Met	
Sodium Intake Managed	
Bracing & Taping Applied	
Sleep Quality (Restful)	

TRIGGERS & OBSERVATIONS

SMALL VICTORIES

- [ ]
- [ ]
- [ ]
- [ ]
- [ ]
- [ ]
- [ ]
- [ ]
- [ ]
- [ ]
- [ ]
- [ ]

Weekly Trackers & Notes

Trackers, triggers, and small victories

DAILY PROTOCOLS & METRICS

Hydration Target Met	
Sodium Intake Managed	
Bracing & Taping Applied	
Sleep Quality (Restful)	

TRIGGERS & OBSERVATIONS

SMALL VICTORIES

- [ ]
- [ ]
- [ ]
- [ ]
- [ ]
- [ ]
- [ ]
- [ ]
- [ ]
- [ ]
- [ ]
- [ ]

Weekly Trackers & Notes

Trackers, triggers, and small victories

DAILY PROTOCOLS & METRICS

Hydration Target Met	
Sodium Intake Managed	
Bracing & Taping Applied	
Sleep Quality (Restful)	

TRIGGERS & OBSERVATIONS

SMALL VICTORIES

- [ ]
- [ ]
- [ ]
- [ ]
- [ ]
- [ ]
- [ ]
- [ ]
- [ ]
- [ ]
- [ ]
- [ ]

Weekly Trackers & Notes

Trackers, triggers, and small victories

DAILY PROTOCOLS & METRICS

Hydration Target Met	
Sodium Intake Managed	
Bracing & Taping Applied	
Sleep Quality (Restful)	

TRIGGERS & OBSERVATIONS

SMALL VICTORIES

- [ ]
- [ ]
- [ ]
- [ ]
- [ ]
- [ ]
- [ ]
- [ ]
- [ ]
- [ ]
- [ ]
- [ ]

Weekly Trackers & Notes

Trackers, triggers, and small victories

DAILY PROTOCOLS & METRICS

Hydration Target Met	
Sodium Intake Managed	
Bracing & Taping Applied	
Sleep Quality (Restful)	

TRIGGERS & OBSERVATIONS

SMALL VICTORIES

- ☐
- ☐
- ☐
- ☐
- ☐
- ☐
- ☐
- ☐
- ☐
- ☐
- ☐
- ☐

Weekly Trackers & Notes

Trackers, triggers, and small victories

DAILY PROTOCOLS & METRICS

Hydration Target Met	
Sodium Intake Managed	
Bracing & Taping Applied	
Sleep Quality (Restful)	

TRIGGERS & OBSERVATIONS

SMALL VICTORIES

- [ ]
- [ ]
- [ ]
- [ ]
- [ ]
- [ ]
- [ ]
- [ ]
- [ ]
- [ ]
- [ ]
- [ ]

Weekly Trackers & Notes

Trackers, triggers, and small victories

DAILY PROTOCOLS & METRICS

Hydration Target Met	
Sodium Intake Managed	
Bracing & Taping Applied	
Sleep Quality (Restful)	

TRIGGERS & OBSERVATIONS

SMALL VICTORIES

- [ ]
- [ ]
- [ ]
- [ ]
- [ ]
- [ ]
- [ ]
- [ ]
- [ ]
- [ ]
- [ ]
- [ ]

Weekly Trackers & Notes

Trackers, triggers, and small victories

DAILY PROTOCOLS & METRICS

Hydration Target Met	
Sodium Intake Managed	
Bracing & Taping Applied	
Sleep Quality (Restful)	

TRIGGERS & OBSERVATIONS

SMALL VICTORIES

- [ ]
- [ ]
- [ ]
- [ ]
- [ ]
- [ ]
- [ ]
- [ ]
- [ ]
- [ ]
- [ ]
- [ ]

Weekly Trackers & Notes

Trackers, triggers, and small victories

DAILY PROTOCOLS & METRICS

Hydration Target Met	
Sodium Intake Managed	
Bracing & Taping Applied	
Sleep Quality (Restful)	

TRIGGERS & OBSERVATIONS

SMALL VICTORIES

- [ ]
- [ ]
- [ ]
- [ ]
- [ ]
- [ ]
- [ ]
- [ ]
- [ ]
- [ ]
- [ ]
- [ ]

Weekly Trackers & Notes

Trackers, triggers, and small victories

DAILY PROTOCOLS & METRICS

Hydration Target Met	
Sodium Intake Managed	
Bracing & Taping Applied	
Sleep Quality (Restful)	

TRIGGERS & OBSERVATIONS

SMALL VICTORIES

- [ ]
- [ ]
- [ ]
- [ ]
- [ ]
- [ ]
- [ ]
- [ ]
- [ ]
- [ ]
- [ ]
- [ ]

Weekly Trackers & Notes

Trackers, triggers, and small victories

DAILY PROTOCOLS & METRICS

Hydration Target Met	
Sodium Intake Managed	
Bracing & Taping Applied	
Sleep Quality (Restful)	

TRIGGERS & OBSERVATIONS

SMALL VICTORIES

- [ ]
- [ ]
- [ ]
- [ ]
- [ ]
- [ ]
- [ ]
- [ ]
- [ ]
- [ ]
- [ ]
- [ ]

Weekly Trackers & Notes

Trackers, triggers, and small victories

DAILY PROTOCOLS & METRICS

Hydration Target Met	
Sodium Intake Managed	
Bracing & Taping Applied	
Sleep Quality (Restful)	

TRIGGERS & OBSERVATIONS

SMALL VICTORIES

- [ ]
- [ ]
- [ ]
- [ ]
- [ ]
- [ ]
- [ ]
- [ ]
- [ ]
- [ ]
- [ ]
- [ ]

Appointment Notes

Prep, vitals, consultation notes, and action plan

Date: ______ **Doctor / Specialty:** ____ **Time:** _____

SYMPTOM SUMMARY & TRIGGERS

ORTHOSTATIC VITALS (DYSAUTONOMIA)

Position / Time	HR (bpm)	Blood Pressure	Symptoms

QUESTIONS TO ASK

- ☐
- ☐
- ☐
- ☐
- ☐
- ☐

CURRENT MEDS & RECENT CHANGES

PHYSICIAN FEEDBACK & CONSULTATION NOTES

ACTIONABLE NEXT STEPS / ORDERS

- ☐
- ☐
- ☐
- ☐

Follow-up Appt: __

Pharmacy / Labs: __

Appointment Notes

Prep, vitals, consultation notes, and action plan

Date: ______ Doctor / Specialty: ____ Time: ____

SYMPTOM SUMMARY & TRIGGERS

ORTHOSTATIC VITALS (DYSAUTONOMIA)

Position / Time	HR (bpm)	Blood Pressure	Symptoms

QUESTIONS TO ASK

- [ ]
- [ ]
- [ ]
- [ ]
- [ ]
- [ ]

CURRENT MEDS & RECENT CHANGES

PHYSICIAN FEEDBACK & CONSULTATION NOTES

ACTIONABLE NEXT STEPS / ORDERS

- [ ]
- [ ]
- [ ]
- [ ]

Follow-up Appt: __

Pharmacy / Labs: __

Appointment Notes

Prep, vitals, consultation notes, and action plan

Date: ______ **Doctor / Specialty:** ____ **Time:** ____

SYMPTOM SUMMARY & TRIGGERS

ORTHOSTATIC VITALS (DYSAUTONOMIA)

Position / Time	HR (bpm)	Blood Pressure	Symptoms

QUESTIONS TO ASK

- [ ]
- [ ]
- [ ]
- [ ]
- [ ]
- [ ]

CURRENT MEDS & RECENT CHANGES

PHYSICIAN FEEDBACK & CONSULTATION NOTES

ACTIONABLE NEXT STEPS / ORDERS

- [ ]
- [ ]
- [ ]
- [ ]

Follow-up Appt: __

Pharmacy / Labs: __

Appointment Notes

Prep, vitals, consultation notes, and action plan

Date: ______ Doctor / Specialty: ____ Time: ____

SYMPTOM SUMMARY & TRIGGERS

ORTHOSTATIC VITALS (DYSAUTONOMIA)

Position / Time	HR (bpm)	Blood Pressure	Symptoms

QUESTIONS TO ASK

- [ ]
- [ ]
- [ ]
- [ ]
- [ ]
- [ ]

CURRENT MEDS & RECENT CHANGES

PHYSICIAN FEEDBACK & CONSULTATION NOTES

ACTIONABLE NEXT STEPS / ORDERS

- [ ]
- [ ]
- [ ]
- [ ]

Follow-up Appt: __

Pharmacy / Labs: __

Appointment Notes

Prep, vitals, consultation notes, and action plan

Date: ______ Doctor / Specialty: ____ Time: _____

SYMPTOM SUMMARY & TRIGGERS

ORTHOSTATIC VITALS (DYSAUTONOMIA)

Position / Time	HR (bpm)	Blood Pressure	Symptoms

QUESTIONS TO ASK

- ☐
- ☐
- ☐
- ☐
- ☐
- ☐

CURRENT MEDS & RECENT CHANGES

PHYSICIAN FEEDBACK & CONSULTATION NOTES

ACTIONABLE NEXT STEPS / ORDERS

- ☐
- ☐
- ☐
- ☐

Follow-up Appt: __

Pharmacy / Labs: __

Appointment Notes

Prep, vitals, consultation notes, and action plan

Date: ______ **Doctor / Specialty:** ____ **Time:** ____

SYMPTOM SUMMARY & TRIGGERS

ORTHOSTATIC VITALS (DYSAUTONOMIA)

Position / Time	HR (bpm)	Blood Pressure	Symptoms

QUESTIONS TO ASK

- [ ]
- [ ]
- [ ]
- [ ]
- [ ]
- [ ]

CURRENT MEDS & RECENT CHANGES

PHYSICIAN FEEDBACK & CONSULTATION NOTES

ACTIONABLE NEXT STEPS / ORDERS

- [ ]
- [ ]
- [ ]
- [ ]

Follow-up Appt: __

Pharmacy / Labs: __

Appointment Notes

Prep, vitals, consultation notes, and action plan

Date: ______ Doctor / Specialty: ____ Time: ______

SYMPTOM SUMMARY & TRIGGERS

ORTHOSTATIC VITALS (DYSAUTONOMIA)

Position / Time	HR (bpm)	Blood Pressure	Symptoms

QUESTIONS TO ASK

- ☐
- ☐
- ☐
- ☐
- ☐
- ☐

CURRENT MEDS & RECENT CHANGES

PHYSICIAN FEEDBACK & CONSULTATION NOTES

ACTIONABLE NEXT STEPS / ORDERS

- ☐
- ☐
- ☐
- ☐

Follow-up Appt: __

Pharmacy / Labs: __

Appointment Notes

Prep, vitals, consultation notes, and action plan

Date: ______ **Doctor / Specialty:** ____ **Time:** ____

SYMPTOM SUMMARY & TRIGGERS

ORTHOSTATIC VITALS (DYSAUTONOMIA)

Position / Time	HR (bpm)	Blood Pressure	Symptoms

QUESTIONS TO ASK

- ☐
- ☐
- ☐
- ☐
- ☐
- ☐

CURRENT MEDS & RECENT CHANGES

PHYSICIAN FEEDBACK & CONSULTATION NOTES

ACTIONABLE NEXT STEPS / ORDERS

- ☐
- ☐
- ☐
- ☐

Follow-up Appt: __

Pharmacy / Labs: __

Appointment Notes

Prep, vitals, consultation notes, and action plan

Date: ______ **Doctor / Specialty:** ____ **Time:** ____

SYMPTOM SUMMARY & TRIGGERS

ORTHOSTATIC VITALS (DYSAUTONOMIA)

Position / Time	HR (bpm)	Blood Pressure	Symptoms

QUESTIONS TO ASK

- [ ]
- [ ]
- [ ]
- [ ]
- [ ]
- [ ]

CURRENT MEDS & RECENT CHANGES

PHYSICIAN FEEDBACK & CONSULTATION NOTES

ACTIONABLE NEXT STEPS / ORDERS

- [ ]
- [ ]
- [ ]
- [ ]

Follow-up Appt: __

Pharmacy / Labs: __

Appointment Notes

Prep, vitals, consultation notes, and action plan

Date: ______ Doctor / Specialty: ____ Time: _____

SYMPTOM SUMMARY & TRIGGERS

ORTHOSTATIC VITALS (DYSAUTONOMIA)

Position / Time	HR (bpm)	Blood Pressure	Symptoms

QUESTIONS TO ASK

- [ ]
- [ ]
- [ ]
- [ ]
- [ ]
- [ ]

CURRENT MEDS & RECENT CHANGES

PHYSICIAN FEEDBACK & CONSULTATION NOTES

ACTIONABLE NEXT STEPS / ORDERS

- [ ]
- [ ]
- [ ]
- [ ]

Follow-up Appt: __

Pharmacy / Labs: __

Appointment Notes

Prep, vitals, consultation notes, and action plan

Date: ______ Doctor / Specialty: ____ Time: ______

SYMPTOM SUMMARY & TRIGGERS

ORTHOSTATIC VITALS (DYSAUTONOMIA)

Position / Time	HR (bpm)	Blood Pressure	Symptoms

QUESTIONS TO ASK

- ☐
- ☐
- ☐
- ☐
- ☐
- ☐

CURRENT MEDS & RECENT CHANGES

PHYSICIAN FEEDBACK & CONSULTATION NOTES

ACTIONABLE NEXT STEPS / ORDERS

- ☐
- ☐
- ☐
- ☐

Follow-up Appt: __

Pharmacy / Labs: __

Appointment Notes

Prep, vitals, consultation notes, and action plan

Date: ______ **Doctor / Specialty:** ____ **Time:** _____

SYMPTOM SUMMARY & TRIGGERS

ORTHOSTATIC VITALS (DYSAUTONOMIA)

Position / Time	HR (bpm)	Blood Pressure	Symptoms

QUESTIONS TO ASK

- [ ]
- [ ]
- [ ]
- [ ]
- [ ]
- [ ]

CURRENT MEDS & RECENT CHANGES

PHYSICIAN FEEDBACK & CONSULTATION NOTES

ACTIONABLE NEXT STEPS / ORDERS

- [ ]
- [ ]
- [ ]
- [ ]

Follow-up Appt: __

Pharmacy / Labs: __

Appointment Notes

Prep, vitals, consultation notes, and action plan

Date: ______ Doctor / Specialty: ____ Time: ____

SYMPTOM SUMMARY & TRIGGERS

ORTHOSTATIC VITALS (DYSAUTONOMIA)

Position / Time	HR (bpm)	Blood Pressure	Symptoms

QUESTIONS TO ASK

- [ ]
- [ ]
- [ ]
- [ ]
- [ ]
- [ ]

CURRENT MEDS & RECENT CHANGES

PHYSICIAN FEEDBACK & CONSULTATION NOTES

ACTIONABLE NEXT STEPS / ORDERS

- [ ]
- [ ]
- [ ]
- [ ]

Follow-up Appt: __

Pharmacy / Labs: __

Appointment Notes

Prep, vitals, consultation notes, and action plan

Date: ______ **Doctor / Specialty:** ____ **Time:** _____

SYMPTOM SUMMARY & TRIGGERS

ORTHOSTATIC VITALS (DYSAUTONOMIA)

Position / Time	HR (bpm)	Blood Pressure	Symptoms

QUESTIONS TO ASK

- [ ]
- [ ]
- [ ]
- [ ]
- [ ]
- [ ]

CURRENT MEDS & RECENT CHANGES

PHYSICIAN FEEDBACK & CONSULTATION NOTES

ACTIONABLE NEXT STEPS / ORDERS

- [ ]
- [ ]
- [ ]
- [ ]

Follow-up Appt: __

Pharmacy / Labs: __

Appointment Notes

Prep, vitals, consultation notes, and action plan

Date: ______ **Doctor / Specialty:** ____ **Time:** ____

SYMPTOM SUMMARY & TRIGGERS

ORTHOSTATIC VITALS (DYSAUTONOMIA)

Position / Time	HR (bpm)	Blood Pressure	Symptoms

QUESTIONS TO ASK

- ☐
- ☐
- ☐
- ☐
- ☐
- ☐

CURRENT MEDS & RECENT CHANGES

PHYSICIAN FEEDBACK & CONSULTATION NOTES

ACTIONABLE NEXT STEPS / ORDERS

- ☐
- ☐
- ☐
- ☐

Follow-up Appt: __

Pharmacy / Labs: __

Flare-Up Protocol

Emergency management for severe pain & dislocation days

Date: ______ PAIN LEVEL **Trigger:** ○○○○○○○○○○ ____________________

RESCUE MEDS & DOSAGES

- ☐ ______
- ☐ ______
- ☐ ______
- ☐ ______
- ☐ ______
- ☐ ______

COMFORT ITEMS (ICE, HEAT, BRACES)

- ☐ ______
- ☐ ______
- ☐ ______
- ☐ ______
- ☐ ______
- ☐ ______

SAFE RESTING POSITIONS

______

______

______

JOINTS AFFECTED / SUBLUXATIONS

______

______

______

TOP 3 IMMEDIATE ACTIONS

1. ______
2. ______
3. ______

SUPPORT CONTACTS

Name / Doctor	Number / Notes

Rest is a vital intervention. Give your body the time and grace it needs to stabilize and heal.

POST-FLARE NOTES (WHAT WORKED, WHAT TO ADJUST)

______

______

______

Flare-Up Protocol

Emergency management for severe pain & dislocation days

Date: _____ **Trigger:** ○ ○ ○ ○ ○ ○ ○ ○ ○ ○ ____________________

RESCUE MEDS & DOSAGES

- ☐ ____________________
- ☐ ____________________
- ☐ ____________________
- ☐ ____________________
- ☐ ____________________
- ☐ ____________________

COMFORT ITEMS (ICE, HEAT, BRACES)

- ☐ ____________________
- ☐ ____________________
- ☐ ____________________
- ☐ ____________________
- ☐ ____________________
- ☐ ____________________

SAFE RESTING POSITIONS

JOINTS AFFECTED / SUBLUXATIONS

TOP 3 IMMEDIATE ACTIONS

1. ____________________
2. ____________________
3. ____________________

SUPPORT CONTACTS

Name / Doctor	Number / Notes

Rest is a vital intervention. Give your body the time and grace it needs to stabilize and heal.

POST-FLARE NOTES (WHAT WORKED, WHAT TO ADJUST)

Therapy Log

Record physical therapy, aids, heat/ice, and their effectiveness

Date: ______ **Primary Focus/Area:** ______ **INITIAL PAIN:** ○○○○○○○○○○

INTERVENTIONS & MODALITIES

Therapy / Modality	Duration / Reps	Settings / Details	Effectiveness (1-10)

OBSERVATIONS & RESULTS

- ☐ Immediate relief
- ☐ Delayed relief
- ☐ Improved mobility/ROM
- ☐ Increased soreness
- ☐ Fatigue
- ☐ No noticeable change

SESSION NOTES (PT EXERCISES, TENS PLACEMENT)

OVERALL RELIEF: ☐☐☐☐☐☐☐☐☐☐

Next Session: ______

ADJUSTMENTS FOR NEXT TIME

Therapy Log

Record physical therapy, aids, heat/ice, and their effectiveness

Date: __________ **Primary Focus/Area:** ____ **INITIAL PAIN:** ○○○○○○○

INTERVENTIONS & MODALITIES

Therapy / Modality	Duration / Reps	Settings / Details	Effectiveness (1-10)

OBSERVATIONS & RESULTS

- ☐ Immediate relief
- ☐ Delayed relief
- ☐ Improved mobility/ROM
- ☐ Increased soreness
- ☐ Fatigue
- ☐ No noticeable change

SESSION NOTES (PT EXERCISES, TENS PLACEMENT)

OVERALL RELIEF: ☐☐☐☐☐☐☐☐☐☐

Next Session: __________

ADJUSTMENTS FOR NEXT TIME

Therapy Log

Record physical therapy, aids, heat/ice, and their effectiveness

Date: ______ **Primary Focus/Area:** ____ **INITIAL PAIN:** ○○○○○○○○○○

INTERVENTIONS & MODALITIES

Therapy / Modality	Duration / Reps	Settings / Details	Effectiveness (1-10)

OBSERVATIONS & RESULTS

- ☐ Immediate relief
- ☐ Delayed relief
- ☐ Improved mobility/ROM
- ☐ Increased soreness
- ☐ Fatigue
- ☐ No noticeable change

SESSION NOTES (PT EXERCISES, TENS PLACEMENT)

OVERALL RELIEF: ☐☐☐☐☐☐☐☐☐☐

Next Session: ________

ADJUSTMENTS FOR NEXT TIME

Therapy Log

Record physical therapy, aids, heat/ice, and their effectiveness

Date: ________ **Primary Focus/Area:** ____ **INITIAL PAIN:** ○○○○○○

INTERVENTIONS & MODALITIES

Therapy / Modality	Duration / Reps	Settings / Details	Effectiveness (1-10)

OBSERVATIONS & RESULTS

- ☐ Immediate relief
- ☐ Delayed relief
- ☐ Improved mobility/ROM
- ☐ Increased soreness
- ☐ Fatigue
- ☐ No noticeable change

SESSION NOTES (PT EXERCISES, TENS PLACEMENT)

OVERALL RELIEF: ☐☐☐☐☐☐☐☐☐☐

Next Session: ________

ADJUSTMENTS FOR NEXT TIME

Therapy Log

Record physical therapy, aids, heat/ice, and their effectiveness

Date: ____________ **Primary Focus/Area:** ____ **INITIAL PAIN:** ○○○○○○○○○○

INTERVENTIONS & MODALITIES

Therapy / Modality	Duration / Reps	Settings / Details	Effectiveness (1-10)

OBSERVATIONS & RESULTS

- ☐ Immediate relief
- ☐ Delayed relief
- ☐ Improved mobility/ROM
- ☐ Increased soreness
- ☐ Fatigue
- ☐ No noticeable change

SESSION NOTES (PT EXERCISES, TENS PLACEMENT)

OVERALL RELIEF: ☐☐☐☐☐☐☐☐☐☐

Next Session: ____________

ADJUSTMENTS FOR NEXT TIME

Therapy Log

Record physical therapy, aids, heat/ice, and their effectiveness

Date: ________ **Primary Focus/Area:** ____ **INITIAL PAIN:** ○○○○○○○

INTERVENTIONS & MODALITIES

Therapy / Modality	Duration / Reps	Settings / Details	Effectiveness (1-10)

OBSERVATIONS & RESULTS

- ☐ Immediate relief
- ☐ Delayed relief
- ☐ Improved mobility/ROM
- ☐ Increased soreness
- ☐ Fatigue
- ☐ No noticeable change

SESSION NOTES (PT EXERCISES, TENS PLACEMENT)

OVERALL RELIEF: ☐☐☐☐☐☐☐☐☐

Next Session: ________

ADJUSTMENTS FOR NEXT TIME

Therapy Log

Record physical therapy, aids, heat/ice, and their effectiveness

Date: ____________ **Primary Focus/Area:** ____ **INITIAL PAIN:** ○○○○○○○○○○

INTERVENTIONS & MODALITIES

Therapy / Modality	Duration / Reps	Settings / Details	Effectiveness (1-10)

OBSERVATIONS & RESULTS

- ☐ Immediate relief
- ☐ Delayed relief
- ☐ Improved mobility/ROM
- ☐ Increased soreness
- ☐ Fatigue
- ☐ No noticeable change

SESSION NOTES (PT EXERCISES, TENS PLACEMENT)

OVERALL RELIEF: ☐☐☐☐☐☐☐☐☐☐

Next Session: ________

ADJUSTMENTS FOR NEXT TIME

Therapy Log

Record physical therapy, aids, heat/ice, and their effectiveness

Date: ________ **Primary Focus/Area:** ____ **INITIAL PAIN:** ○○○○○○○

INTERVENTIONS & MODALITIES

Therapy / Modality	Duration / Reps	Settings / Details	Effectiveness (1-10)

OBSERVATIONS & RESULTS

- ☐ Immediate relief
- ☐ Delayed relief
- ☐ Improved mobility/ROM
- ☐ Increased soreness
- ☐ Fatigue
- ☐ No noticeable change

SESSION NOTES (PT EXERCISES, TENS PLACEMENT)

OVERALL RELIEF: ☐☐☐☐☐☐☐☐☐☐

Next Session: ________

ADJUSTMENTS FOR NEXT TIME

Monthly Reflection

Treatments, triggers, and pacing review

Month / Year: _____ SEVERITY: ○○○○○ ENERGY: ☆☆☆☆☆

TREATMENT & RELIEF REVIEW

Treatment / Therapy	Freq / Dose	Relief (1-10)	Notes / Side Effects

NEWLY DISCOVERED TRIGGERS

SYMPTOM PATTERNS & FLARE-UPS

PACING STRATEGIES FOR NEXT MONTH

BOUNDARIES & LIMITS TO SET

- ☐
- ☐
- ☐
- ☐
- ☐

QUESTIONS FOR HEALTHCARE TEAM

ADJUSTMENTS & SELF-COMPASSION

Monthly Reflection

Treatments, triggers, and pacing review

Month / Year: _____ **SEVERITY:** ○○○○○ **ENERGY:** ☆☆☆☆☆

TREATMENT & RELIEF REVIEW

Treatment / Therapy	Freq / Dose	Relief (1-10)	Notes / Side Effects

NEWLY DISCOVERED TRIGGERS

SYMPTOM PATTERNS & FLARE-UPS

PACING STRATEGIES FOR NEXT MONTH

BOUNDARIES & LIMITS TO SET

- ☐ ____________________
- ☐ ____________________
- ☐ ____________________
- ☐ ____________________
- ☐ ____________________

QUESTIONS FOR HEALTHCARE TEAM

ADJUSTMENTS & SELF-COMPASSION

Monthly Reflection

Treatments, triggers, and pacing review

Month / Year: _____ SEVERITY: ○○○○○ ENERGY: ☆☆☆☆☆

TREATMENT & RELIEF REVIEW

Treatment / Therapy	Freq / Dose	Relief (1-10)	Notes / Side Effects

NEWLY DISCOVERED TRIGGERS

SYMPTOM PATTERNS & FLARE-UPS

PACING STRATEGIES FOR NEXT MONTH

BOUNDARIES & LIMITS TO SET

- ☐
- ☐
- ☐
- ☐
- ☐

QUESTIONS FOR HEALTHCARE TEAM

ADJUSTMENTS & SELF-COMPASSION

Monthly Reflection

Treatments, triggers, and pacing review

Month / Year: _____ **SEVERITY:** ○○○○○ **ENERGY:** ☆☆☆☆☆

TREATMENT & RELIEF REVIEW

Treatment / Therapy	Freq / Dose	Relief (1-10)	Notes / Side Effects

NEWLY DISCOVERED TRIGGERS

SYMPTOM PATTERNS & FLARE-UPS

PACING STRATEGIES FOR NEXT MONTH

BOUNDARIES & LIMITS TO SET

- ☐
- ☐
- ☐
- ☐
- ☐

QUESTIONS FOR HEALTHCARE TEAM

ADJUSTMENTS & SELF-COMPASSION

Monthly Reflection

Treatments, triggers, and pacing review

Month / Year: _____ **SEVERITY:** ○○○○○ **ENERGY:** ☆☆☆☆☆

TREATMENT & RELIEF REVIEW

Treatment / Therapy	Freq / Dose	Relief (1-10)	Notes / Side Effects

NEWLY DISCOVERED TRIGGERS

SYMPTOM PATTERNS & FLARE-UPS

PACING STRATEGIES FOR NEXT MONTH

BOUNDARIES & LIMITS TO SET

- [ ]
- [ ]
- [ ]
- [ ]
- [ ]

QUESTIONS FOR HEALTHCARE TEAM

ADJUSTMENTS & SELF-COMPASSION

Monthly Reflection

Treatments, triggers, and pacing review

Month / Year: _____ SEVERITY: ○○○○○ ENERGY: ☆☆☆☆☆

TREATMENT & RELIEF REVIEW

Treatment / Therapy	Freq / Dose	Relief (1-10)	Notes / Side Effects

NEWLY DISCOVERED TRIGGERS

SYMPTOM PATTERNS & FLARE-UPS

PACING STRATEGIES FOR NEXT MONTH

BOUNDARIES & LIMITS TO SET

- ☐
- ☐
- ☐
- ☐
- ☐

QUESTIONS FOR HEALTHCARE TEAM

ADJUSTMENTS & SELF-COMPASSION

6-Month Health Review

Trends, resilience, and preparation for the next specialist visit

Period Covered: _____ **Specialist/Doc:** ______ **Appt Date:** ______

KEY DATA POINTS & METRICS (6-MONTH TREND)

Metric / Symptom	Start Value	Peak / Low	Current Value	Key Notes

MAJOR HEALTH TRENDS & OBSERVATIONS

TREATMENT & MEDICATION EFFICACY

CELEBRATING RESILIENCE: CHALLENGES OVERCOME & PERSONAL WINS

QUESTIONS & CONCERNS FOR SPECIALIST

- [ ]
- [ ]
- [ ]
- [ ]
- [ ]
- [ ]

ACTION PLAN & GOALS FOR NEXT 6 MONTHS

EDS: because my body likes to keep things interesting.

Date: ________________ **Mood:** ________________

WHAT THIS QUOTE MEANS TO ME RIGHT NOW

WHEN HAVE I LIVED THIS — OR FAILED TO?

HOW WILL I ACT ON THIS TODAY?

One word I want to carry: ________________

Person I will share this with: ________________

My joints missed the memo about staying in place.

Date: ________________ **Mood:** ________________

WHAT THIS QUOTE MEANS TO ME RIGHT NOW

WHEN HAVE I LIVED THIS — OR FAILED TO?

HOW WILL I ACT ON THIS TODAY?

One word I want to carry: ________________

Person I will share this with: ________________

I don't fall apart. I simply come with extra moving parts.

Date: ________________ **Mood:** ________________

WHAT THIS QUOTE MEANS TO ME RIGHT NOW

WHEN HAVE I LIVED THIS — OR FAILED TO?

HOW WILL I ACT ON THIS TODAY?

One word I want to carry: ________________

Person I will share this with: ________________

My body believes stability is optional.

Date: ________________ **Mood:** ________________

WHAT THIS QUOTE MEANS TO ME RIGHT NOW

WHEN HAVE I LIVED THIS — OR FAILED TO?

HOW WILL I ACT ON THIS TODAY?

One word I want to carry: ____________________

Person I will share this with: ____________________

I'm held together by determination, hope, and kinesiology tape.

Date: ________________ **Mood:** ______________

WHAT THIS QUOTE MEANS TO ME RIGHT NOW

WHEN HAVE I LIVED THIS — OR FAILED TO?

HOW WILL I ACT ON THIS TODAY?

One word I want to carry: ________________

Person I will share this with: ______________

My joints have a mind of their own.

Date: ________________ **Mood:** _______________

WHAT THIS QUOTE MEANS TO ME RIGHT NOW

WHEN HAVE I LIVED THIS — OR FAILED TO?

HOW WILL I ACT ON THIS TODAY?

One word I want to carry: ________________

Person I will share this with: ________________

I don't need a weather app. My body already knows.

Date: ________________ **Mood:** ________________

WHAT THIS QUOTE MEANS TO ME RIGHT NOW

WHEN HAVE I LIVED THIS — OR FAILED TO?

HOW WILL I ACT ON THIS TODAY?

One word I want to carry: ________________

Person I will share this with: ________________

Every day is a new episode of 'What Hurts Today?'

Date: ________________ **Mood:** _______________

WHAT THIS QUOTE MEANS TO ME RIGHT NOW

WHEN HAVE I LIVED THIS — OR FAILED TO?

HOW WILL I ACT ON THIS TODAY?

One word I want to carry: ____________________

Person I will share this with: ___________________

My body likes surprise plot twists.

Date: ________________ **Mood:** _______________

WHAT THIS QUOTE MEANS TO ME RIGHT NOW

WHEN HAVE I LIVED THIS — OR FAILED TO?

HOW WILL I ACT ON THIS TODAY?

One word I want to carry: ____________________

Person I will share this with: ____________________

I'm basically a professional at adapting.

Date: ________________ **Mood:** ________________

WHAT THIS QUOTE MEANS TO ME RIGHT NOW

WHEN HAVE I LIVED THIS — OR FAILED TO?

HOW WILL I ACT ON THIS TODAY?

One word I want to carry: ________________

Person I will share this with: ________________

Some people stretch. My joints volunteer.

Date: ________________ **Mood:** _______________

WHAT THIS QUOTE MEANS TO ME RIGHT NOW

WHEN HAVE I LIVED THIS — OR FAILED TO?

HOW WILL I ACT ON THIS TODAY?

One word I want to carry: ________________

Person I will share this with: ________________

I've mastered the art of laughing through flare days.

Date: ________________ **Mood:** ________________

WHAT THIS QUOTE MEANS TO ME RIGHT NOW

WHEN HAVE I LIVED THIS — OR FAILED TO?

HOW WILL I ACT ON THIS TODAY?

One word I want to carry: ________________

Person I will share this with: ________________

My body may be unpredictable, but my spirit isn't.

Date: ________________ **Mood:** ________________

WHAT THIS QUOTE MEANS TO ME RIGHT NOW

WHEN HAVE I LIVED THIS — OR FAILED TO?

HOW WILL I ACT ON THIS TODAY?

One word I want to carry: ________________

Person I will share this with: ________________

Rest is part of my strength, not a sign of weakness.

Date: ________________ **Mood:** ________________

WHAT THIS QUOTE MEANS TO ME RIGHT NOW

WHEN HAVE I LIVED THIS — OR FAILED TO?

HOW WILL I ACT ON THIS TODAY?

One word I want to carry: ________________

Person I will share this with: ________________

My superpower is getting back up, every single time.

Date: ________________ **Mood:** ________________

WHAT THIS QUOTE MEANS TO ME RIGHT NOW

WHEN HAVE I LIVED THIS — OR FAILED TO?

HOW WILL I ACT ON THIS TODAY?

One word I want to carry: ________________

Person I will share this with: ________________

My body writes stories I never planned to tell.

Date: ________________ **Mood:** ________________

WHAT THIS QUOTE MEANS TO ME RIGHT NOW

WHEN HAVE I LIVED THIS — OR FAILED TO?

HOW WILL I ACT ON THIS TODAY?

One word I want to carry: ________________

Person I will share this with: ________________

I may move a little slower, but I never stop moving forward.

Date: ________________ **Mood:** ________________

WHAT THIS QUOTE MEANS TO ME RIGHT NOW

WHEN HAVE I LIVED THIS — OR FAILED TO?

HOW WILL I ACT ON THIS TODAY?

One word I want to carry: ________________

Person I will share this with: ________________

My joints enjoy making every day an adventure.

Date: ________________ **Mood:** ______________

WHAT THIS QUOTE MEANS TO ME RIGHT NOW

WHEN HAVE I LIVED THIS — OR FAILED TO?

HOW WILL I ACT ON THIS TODAY?

One word I want to carry: ________________

Person I will share this with: ________________

I've become an expert in celebrating small victories.

Date: ________________ **Mood:** ________________

WHAT THIS QUOTE MEANS TO ME RIGHT NOW

WHEN HAVE I LIVED THIS — OR FAILED TO?

HOW WILL I ACT ON THIS TODAY?

One word I want to carry: ________________

Person I will share this with: ________________

Life with EDS has made me stronger than I ever imagined.

Date: ________________ **Mood:** ________________

WHAT THIS QUOTE MEANS TO ME RIGHT NOW

WHEN HAVE I LIVED THIS — OR FAILED TO?

HOW WILL I ACT ON THIS TODAY?

One word I want to carry: ________________

Person I will share this with: ________________

My body loves surprises. I prefer coffee.

Date: ________________ **Mood:** _______________

WHAT THIS QUOTE MEANS TO ME RIGHT NOW

WHEN HAVE I LIVED THIS — OR FAILED TO?

HOW WILL I ACT ON THIS TODAY?

One word I want to carry: ____________________

Person I will share this with: __________________

I don't give up. I simply recharge.

Date: ________________ **Mood:** ________________

WHAT THIS QUOTE MEANS TO ME RIGHT NOW

WHEN HAVE I LIVED THIS — OR FAILED TO?

HOW WILL I ACT ON THIS TODAY?

One word I want to carry: ________________

Person I will share this with: ________________

My resilience is stronger than my symptoms.

Date: ________________ **Mood:** ________________

WHAT THIS QUOTE MEANS TO ME RIGHT NOW

WHEN HAVE I LIVED THIS — OR FAILED TO?

HOW WILL I ACT ON THIS TODAY?

One word I want to carry: ________________

Person I will share this with: ________________

Some days I conquer mountains. Other days I conquer getting out of bed.

Date: ________________ **Mood:** ________________

WHAT THIS QUOTE MEANS TO ME RIGHT NOW

WHEN HAVE I LIVED THIS — OR FAILED TO?

HOW WILL I ACT ON THIS TODAY?

One word I want to carry: ________________

Person I will share this with: ________________

I've learned that progress doesn't have to be perfect.

Date: ________________ **Mood:** ________________

WHAT THIS QUOTE MEANS TO ME RIGHT NOW

WHEN HAVE I LIVED THIS — OR FAILED TO?

HOW WILL I ACT ON THIS TODAY?

One word I want to carry: ________________

Person I will share this with: ________________

My body bends. My determination never does.

Date: ________________ **Mood:** ________________

WHAT THIS QUOTE MEANS TO ME RIGHT NOW

WHEN HAVE I LIVED THIS — OR FAILED TO?

HOW WILL I ACT ON THIS TODAY?

One word I want to carry: ________________

Person I will share this with: ________________

Strength isn't measured by perfect joints.

Date: ________________ **Mood:** _______________

WHAT THIS QUOTE MEANS TO ME RIGHT NOW

WHEN HAVE I LIVED THIS — OR FAILED TO?

HOW WILL I ACT ON THIS TODAY?

One word I want to carry: ____________________

Person I will share this with: __________________

I may have EDS, but EDS doesn't have me.

Date: ________________ Mood: ________________

WHAT THIS QUOTE MEANS TO ME RIGHT NOW

WHEN HAVE I LIVED THIS — OR FAILED TO?

HOW WILL I ACT ON THIS TODAY?

One word I want to carry: ________________

Person I will share this with: ________________

Every flare reminds me how resilient I truly am.

Date: ________________ **Mood:** ______________

WHAT THIS QUOTE MEANS TO ME RIGHT NOW

WHEN HAVE I LIVED THIS — OR FAILED TO?

HOW WILL I ACT ON THIS TODAY?

One word I want to carry: ________________

Person I will share this with: ________________

I'm proof that courage comes in many forms.

Date: ________________ **Mood:** _______________

WHAT THIS QUOTE MEANS TO ME RIGHT NOW

WHEN HAVE I LIVED THIS — OR FAILED TO?

HOW WILL I ACT ON THIS TODAY?

One word I want to carry: ____________________

Person I will share this with: ________________

www.ingramcontent.com/pod-product-compliance
Lightning Source LLC
Chambersburg PA
CBHW050529240926
51846CB00003B/751